CHAIR WORKOUT

FOR SENIORS

Comprehensive, Easy-To-Follow, Low-Impact Exercise Routines For Strength, Flexibility, And Balance To Enhance Mobility And Well-Being

ROBERT LUGO

CHAPTER 1
Introduction To Chair Workouts

Chair workouts offer a unique and accessible way for seniors to engage in physical activity and improve their overall health and well-being.

These workouts are designed to be performed while seated or using a chair for support, making them suitable for individuals with limited mobility or those who prefer a low-impact exercise option.

The concept of chair workouts has gained popularity in recent years due to their effectiveness in promoting strength, flexibility, and cardiovascular health without putting excessive strain on joints or muscles. Seniors can benefit greatly from incorporating chair exercises into their daily routine, helping them maintain independence, prevent falls, and enhance their quality of life.

Importance of Exercise for Seniors:

Seniors who want to preserve their physical and mental well-being as they age must engage in regular exercise.

As individuals grow older, they may experience a decline in muscle mass, flexibility, and overall fitness level. Engaging in regular physical activity, such as chair workouts, can help counteract these effects and improve functional abilities.

Exercise also plays a vital role in managing chronic conditions commonly associated with aging, such as arthritis, osteoporosis, diabetes, and heart disease. Additionally, staying active can boost mood, cognitive function, and overall well-being, promoting a higher quality of life for seniors.

Benefits of Chair Workouts:

Chair workouts offer a wide range of benefits for seniors, making them an ideal choice for staying active and healthy.

One of the primary benefits is improved strength and muscle tone, particularly in the lower body, core, and upper extremities.

By incorporating resistance exercises using the chair as a prop, seniors can effectively target various muscle groups and enhance their overall physical strength. Chair workouts also contribute to better balance and stability, reducing the risk of falls and injuries, which is especially important for older adults. Additionally, these exercises promote flexibility, joint mobility, and cardiovascular fitness, supporting overall functional independence and longevity.

Synopsis of Safety Considerations:

When engaging in chair workouts, safety considerations are paramount to ensure a positive and injury-free experience for seniors. It's essential to choose exercises that are appropriate for the individual's fitness level and physical capabilities. Beginners should start with gentle movements and gradually progress to more challenging exercises as they build strength and confidence. Proper posture and alignment are also crucial during chair workouts to prevent strain or discomfort. Seniors should be encouraged to listen to their bodies, avoid overexertion, and take breaks as needed. Additionally, maintaining a safe workout environment, free from hazards or obstacles, is essential for injury prevention.

Setting Up a Safe Workout Space:

Creating a safe workout space is essential for seniors to feel comfortable and confident during chair workouts. Start by selecting a sturdy and stable chair that provides adequate support for exercises. Ideally, the chair should have a backrest and armrests for added stability. Place the chair on a non-slip surface to prevent it from sliding or moving during workouts.

Ensure that the surrounding area is clear of clutter or obstacles that could pose a tripping hazard. Adequate lighting is also important to ensure visibility and safety during exercise sessions. Seniors should have access to water and any necessary equipment, such as resistance bands or light weights, within reach. By setting up a safe and functional workout space, seniors can focus on their exercises without worrying about potential risks or accidents.

CHAPTER 2
Understanding Senior Fitness

Seniors, typically defined as individuals aged 65 and older, experience a range of physical changes that can significantly impact their fitness levels and overall well-being. Understanding senior fitness entails recognizing these changes and tailoring workout programs to meet the unique needs of older adults.

One of the primary considerations in senior fitness is the gradual decline in muscle mass and strength, known as sarcopenia. This age-related phenomenon affects various muscle groups, especially those essential for mobility and daily activities. Additionally, seniors may experience reduced flexibility and joint stiffness, making movements more challenging and increasing the risk of injuries. Understanding these physiological changes is crucial for designing effective and safe chair workouts for seniors.

Common Age-Related Physical Changes:

Age-related physical changes encompass a spectrum of alterations that impact seniors' physical abilities and health. These changes include decreased bone density, which increases the risk of fractures and osteoporosis.

Joint degeneration, such as arthritis, can lead to pain and limited range of motion, affecting mobility and exercise tolerance. Moreover, age-related declines in cardiovascular function, including reduced aerobic capacity and slower heart rate recovery, necessitate careful consideration in workout planning for seniors.

Assessing Individual Fitness Levels:

Assessing seniors' fitness levels is a foundational step in designing personalized chair workouts. Various assessment tools and techniques can be used to evaluate seniors' physical capabilities, including strength tests, flexibility assessments, balance tests, and cardiovascular fitness evaluations.

These assessments help identify strengths, areas for improvement, and any existing medical conditions that may influence workout programming.

Goals and Expectations for Chair Workouts:

Setting realistic goals and managing expectations are essential aspects of chair workouts for seniors. Goals may include improving strength, flexibility, balance, cardiovascular endurance, and overall functional abilities.

However, it's crucial to align these goals with seniors' abilities and limitations, focusing on gradual progress and consistent effort. Managing expectations involves understanding that fitness improvements may take time and that individual responses to exercise vary based on factors such as age, health status, and fitness background.

Medical advice and assessments play a pivotal role in ensuring the safety and efficacy of chair workouts for seniors. Consulting healthcare professionals, such as physicians, physical therapists, and exercise physiologists, helps identify any contraindications or specific considerations for exercise programming.

Medical assessments, including blood pressure monitoring, medication reviews, and health history evaluations, provide valuable insights for tailoring workouts and addressing potential health risks during exercise sessions.

Integrating medical advice and assessments into chair workouts promotes a holistic approach to senior fitness, focusing on both physical improvements and overall health management.

CHAPTER 3
Warm-Up And Cool-Down Techniques

In chair workouts for seniors, warm-up and cool-down techniques play a crucial role in enhancing the effectiveness and safety of exercise sessions. The concept of warm-up encompasses a series of activities designed to prepare the body for physical exertion. It involves gentle movements that gradually increase heart rate, improve blood circulation, and activate muscles, ligaments, and joints. A well-structured warm-up routine not only reduces the risk of injury but also enhances overall performance during the workout.

The importance of warming up cannot be overstated, especially for seniors. As individuals age, their bodies may require more time and care to prepare for physical activity. A proper warm-up routine helps seniors to gradually transition from a resting state to an active one, minimizing the stress on the cardiovascular system and muscles.

It also helps to lubricate joints, improve flexibility, and enhance coordination, making movements smoother and more controlled.

Gentle stretching routines are an integral part of warm-up sessions in chair workouts for seniors. These stretching exercises focus on improving flexibility, range of motion, and muscle elasticity. They target major muscle groups, such as the legs, arms, shoulders, and back, promoting better mobility and reducing the risk of strains or muscle pulls. Gentle stretching also helps seniors maintain joint health and prevent stiffness, which is common with age-related changes in connective tissues.

Breathing exercises are another essential component of warm-up routines for seniors. Proper breathing techniques not only oxygenate the body but also help seniors to relax, focus, and maintain a steady rhythm during exercise. Deep breathing exercises, such as diaphragmatic breathing or belly breathing, can reduce stress, improve lung capacity, and enhance overall respiratory function. Incorporating breathing exercises into chair workouts encourages seniors to engage in mindful breathing, which supports their physical and mental well-being.

Cool-down strategies are equally important in chair workouts for seniors. The cool-down phase allows the body to gradually return to a resting state after exercise, preventing sudden drops in blood pressure and helping to dissipate accumulated metabolic byproducts, such as lactic acid. Cooling down also promotes muscle recovery, reduces the risk of post-exercise soreness, and enhances flexibility. Common cool-down techniques include gentle stretching, slow-paced movements, and relaxation exercises aimed at calming the mind and body.

warm-up and cool-down techniques are fundamental aspects of chair workouts for seniors. They provide essential preparation before exercise and aid in the recovery process afterward. Incorporating gentle stretching routines, breathing exercises, and effective cool-down strategies not only enhances the physical benefits of exercise but also promotes a sense of well-being and longevity in senior fitness programs.

CHAPTER 4
Upper Body Chair Exercises

Upper-body chair exercises for seniors offer a range of benefits, aiding in maintaining strength, mobility, and overall well-being.

These exercises are tailored to suit the needs of seniors who may have limitations in standing or engaging in high-impact activities. Let's delve into each exercise to understand their mechanics and advantages.

Seated arm raises are a fundamental upper body exercise that targets the shoulders and arms. This exercise involves sitting upright in a chair with feet flat on the floor and arms at your sides.

Slowly raise both arms straight out to the sides until they are parallel to the floor, then lower them back down. This movement helps improve shoulder flexibility and strength, benefiting daily activities like reaching overhead or lifting light objects.

Chair push-ups are modified push-ups that provide a safe yet effective way to strengthen the chest, shoulders, and arms. To perform chair push-ups, sit on the edge of a sturdy chair with hands placed on the seat beside your hips.

Walk your feet forward until your knees are bent at a 90-degree angle. Lower your body towards the chair by bending your elbows, then push back up to the starting position. This exercise builds upper body strength without the intensity of traditional push-ups.

Shoulder presses are excellent for targeting the deltoid muscles in the shoulders. Sit tall in a chair with a sturdy backrest and hold dumbbells or resistance bands in each hand at shoulder height. Press the weights overhead until your arms are fully extended, then lower them back down to shoulder level. This exercise helps improve shoulder stability and is beneficial for tasks requiring overhead reaching or lifting.

Bicep curls focus on strengthening the biceps, essential for activities like lifting groceries or carrying objects. Sit comfortably in a chair with a straight back and hold dumbbells at your sides with palms facing forward. Keeping your elbows close to your body, curl the weights towards your shoulders, then lower them back down with control. Bicep curls enhance arm strength and can contribute to better functional abilities in daily life.

Tricep extensions target the triceps, located at the back of the upper arms, crucial for pushing movements and arm stability. Sit upright in a chair and hold a dumbbell with both hands overhead. Lower the weight behind your head by bending your elbows, then extend your arms to lift the weight back up. Tricep extensions strengthen the back of the arms, aiding in activities like pushing oneself up from a seated position or lifting heavier objects safely.

Incorporating these upper-body chair exercises into a senior fitness routine promotes muscle strength, joint flexibility, and overall physical independence. Consistency and proper form are key to maximizing the benefits of these exercises while minimizing the risk of injury. Encourage seniors to start with light weights and gradually increase resistance as they gain strength and confidence. Regular participation in these exercises can contribute to a healthier, more active lifestyle for seniors.

CHAPTER 5
Lower Body Chair Exercises

Chair workouts offer a viable and effective means for seniors to maintain lower body strength, flexibility, and mobility. These exercises can be performed safely and comfortably while seated, minimizing the risk of falls and injuries.

This comprehensive examination delves into five crucial lower-body chair exercises: Seated Leg Lifts, Chair Squats, Calf Raises, Hamstring Curls, and Ankle Rotations. Each exercise is explored in depth, focusing on proper technique, muscle engagement, benefits, and practical tips to optimize their effectiveness.

Seated Leg Lifts are a foundational exercise in chair workouts for seniors, targeting the quadriceps, hip flexors, and core muscles.

To perform a Seated Leg Lift, one should sit comfortably in a sturdy chair with their back straight and feet flat on the floor.

The exercise begins with the individual slowly lifting one leg to extend it straight out in front, ensuring that the thigh muscles remain engaged throughout the movement. Holding this position briefly before lowering the leg back down enhances muscle activation. Repeating this motion for multiple repetitions on each leg can significantly improve lower body strength and stability.

The primary muscles involved in Seated Leg Lifts include the quadriceps, which are responsible for extending the knee, and the hip flexors, which facilitate the lifting of the leg. Additionally, the core muscles are engaged to maintain proper posture and balance. This exercise is particularly beneficial for seniors as it helps to enhance mobility, making daily activities such as walking and climbing stairs easier. It also aids in maintaining joint health by promoting flexibility and reducing stiffness in the hip and knee joints.

Chair Squats are another essential exercise in chair-based workouts, providing a functional movement pattern that mimics the act of standing up from a seated position. This exercise targets the glutes, quadriceps, hamstrings, and core muscles. To perform Chair Squats, one should start by sitting at the edge of the chair with feet shoulder-width apart and arms either crossed over the chest or extended forward for balance. The movement begins by leaning slightly forward from the hips, then pressing through the heels to stand up, keeping the back straight and core engaged. Lowering back down to a seated position with control completes one repetition.

Chair Squats offer numerous benefits, including improved leg strength, enhanced balance, and better coordination. For seniors, this exercise is particularly advantageous as it replicates a common daily activity, thereby improving functional independence. The gluteal muscles, which are crucial for hip extension and stability, are heavily involved in this exercise.

Strengthening these muscles can alleviate lower back pain and enhance overall posture.

Moreover, Chair Squats help in maintaining bone density, which is vital for preventing osteoporosis in older adults.

Calf Raises are an excellent exercise for strengthening the calf muscles and improving ankle stability. This exercise is performed by sitting in a chair with feet flat on the floor and knees bent at a 90-degree angle.

The individual then raises their heels off the ground, lifting as high as possible while keeping the toes and balls of the feet in contact with the floor. Holding the raised position briefly before lowering the heels back down completes one repetition.

The primary muscles targeted by Calf Raises are the gastrocnemius and soleus muscles of the calf. Strengthening these muscles is essential for activities that require pushing off the toes, such as walking, running, and climbing stairs.

For seniors, strong calf muscles can significantly reduce the risk of falls by improving balance and proprioception. Additionally, Calf Raises promote better circulation in the lower legs, which can help prevent venous insufficiency and reduce swelling.

Hamstring Curls, when adapted for chair workouts, involves engaging the muscles at the back of the thigh. This exercise can be performed by sitting in a chair with the legs extended forward and feet flat on the floor.

The individual then bends one knee, bringing the heel towards the chair's seat while keeping the thigh stationary. Holding the contracted position briefly before returning the foot to the floor completes one repetition.

The hamstring muscles, comprising the biceps femoris, semitendinosus, and semimembranosus, are crucial for knee flexion and hip extension.

Strengthening these muscles through Hamstring Curls can improve gait and enhance overall leg strength.

For seniors, strong hamstrings can help prevent muscle imbalances that lead to knee and hip pain. This exercise also contributes to better posture by supporting the lower back and reducing strain on the spine.

Ankle Rotations are a simple yet effective exercise to enhance ankle flexibility and prevent stiffness. To perform Ankle Rotations, one should sit in a chair with their back straight and feet off the floor. The exercise involves rotating the ankle in a circular motion, first clockwise and then counterclockwise, ensuring that the movement is controlled and deliberate.

The primary muscles and tendons involved in Ankle Rotations include the tibialis anterior, peroneals, and the Achilles tendon. This exercise is particularly beneficial for seniors as it helps maintain joint mobility and flexibility, which are crucial for activities that involve ankle movement, such as walking and balancing.

Regular Ankle Rotations can also prevent conditions such as ankle sprains and improve overall foot health.

Integrating these lower-body chair exercises into a regular fitness routine can significantly enhance the physical well-being of seniors. Seated Leg Lifts, Chair Squats, Calf Raises, Hamstring Curls, and Ankle Rotations each offer unique benefits that contribute to improved strength, flexibility, and balance. By understanding the proper techniques and muscle engagement for these exercises, seniors can perform them safely and effectively, thereby promoting long-term health and functional independence.

CHAPTER 6
Core Strengthening Chair Exercises

In the realm of chair workouts for seniors, core strengthening is a fundamental aspect that contributes significantly to overall fitness and mobility. Core strength refers to the muscles of the abdomen, lower back, and pelvis, which play a crucial role in maintaining posture, balance, and stability.

For seniors, maintaining a strong core is especially important as it supports everyday activities, reduces the risk of falls, and improves overall quality of life. In this section, we delve into core strengthening chair exercises tailored specifically for seniors, focusing on techniques, benefits, and safety considerations.

Seated Abdominal Twists are an effective way to engage the core muscles while seated comfortably in a chair.

This exercise targets the obliques and abdominals, promoting flexibility and strength in the torso.

To perform seated abdominal twists, seniors can sit upright with feet flat on the floor, hold onto the sides of the chair for support, and slowly twist their upper body to the right, then return to the center and repeat on the left side.

This gentle yet impactful movement helps seniors improve spinal mobility and core stability over time.

Chair Leg Raises offer a low-impact yet beneficial way to strengthen the core and lower body muscles. Seniors can sit tall in a chair with hands resting on the sides, then lift one leg straight out in front of them, hold it for a few seconds, and lower it back down.

This exercise targets the hip flexors, quadriceps, and core muscles, aiding in improving balance and leg strength. Variations can include lifting both legs simultaneously or adding ankle weights for increased resistance, depending on individual fitness levels.

Seated Side Bends are another excellent addition to core strengthening chair exercises for seniors. This exercise focuses on the oblique muscles, which are vital for lateral stability and spinal support.

Seniors can sit with feet flat on the floor, raise one arm overhead, and gently lean to the side, aiming to feel a stretch along the opposite side of the torso. By incorporating seated side bends into their routine, seniors can enhance flexibility, posture, and overall core strength.

Pelvic Tilts are simple yet effective chair exercises that target the deep abdominal muscles and promote pelvic stability. Seniors can sit comfortably with feet flat on the floor and hands on the hips, then gently tilt the pelvis forward, arching the lower back slightly, and then tilt it backward, rounding the lower back.

This controlled movement helps seniors strengthen their pelvic floor muscles, improve posture, and alleviate lower back discomfort often associated with age-related changes.

Stability Ball Exercises, although not performed directly on a chair, can be adapted for seniors by using a stability ball while seated. Stability balls provide an unstable surface, engaging core muscles and promoting balance and coordination.

Seniors can perform exercises such as seated ball rotations, ball marches, or ball passes to enhance core strength, stability, and overall fitness. Safety precautions should be taken, ensuring the ball is properly inflated and placed on a non-slip surface.

core strengthening chair exercises offer seniors a safe and effective way to improve core stability, posture, and overall functional fitness.

By incorporating exercises like seated abdominal twists, chair leg raises, seated side bends, pelvic tilts, and adapting stability ball exercises, seniors can enjoy the benefits of a stronger core, enhanced balance, and increased confidence in daily activities. It's essential to start slowly, listen to your body, and consult with a healthcare professional before beginning any new exercise routine.

CHAPTER 7
Cardiovascular Chair Exercises

Cardiovascular Chair Exercises involve a series of movements designed to improve cardiovascular health while minimizing impact on the joints. These exercises are particularly beneficial for seniors as they provide a way to enhance heart health, increase endurance, and improve overall physical fitness without the need for standing or high-impact activities.

These exercises are performed while seated, making them accessible to individuals with varying levels of mobility and fitness. They can be easily adapted to suit individual capabilities, ensuring that everyone can participate regardless of their physical limitations.

By incorporating rhythmic movements and steady pacing, these exercises help elevate the heart rate, thereby promoting cardiovascular endurance.

The effectiveness of Cardiovascular Chair Exercises lies in their ability to engage multiple muscle groups simultaneously, fostering improved circulation and enhanced metabolic function. These exercises typically include movements that mimic traditional aerobic activities, such as marching, arm swings, and leg lifts but are adapted to be performed from a seated position.

This approach not only provides cardiovascular benefits but also helps improve muscle tone and coordination.

One of the key advantages of Cardiovascular Chair Exercises is their versatility. They can be modified to accommodate different fitness levels and can be performed in various settings, from the comfort of one's home to group exercise classes. This adaptability makes them an ideal choice for seniors seeking to maintain an active lifestyle without the risks associated with high-impact workouts.

Incorporating these exercises into a regular fitness routine can lead to significant health improvements. Consistent practice can help reduce the risk of cardiovascular diseases, enhance respiratory function, and improve overall stamina. Additionally, these exercises can contribute to better mental health by reducing stress and promoting a sense of well-being.

Marching in Place is a fundamental component of Cardiovascular Chair Exercises. This activity involves lifting the knees alternately while keeping the upper body stable and engaging the core muscles. By mimicking the motion of walking or marching, this exercise helps elevate the heart rate and improve circulation without the need for weight-bearing movements.

The simplicity of Marching in Place makes it an excellent starting point for seniors new to exercise or those with limited mobility. It requires no special equipment and can be performed in a small space, making it accessible to virtually anyone. Moreover, this exercise can be easily adjusted to match individual fitness levels by varying the speed and height of the knee lifts.

In addition to its cardiovascular benefits, Marching in Place also aids in improving coordination and balance. By engaging the lower body muscles, this exercise helps strengthen the legs and core, which are crucial for maintaining stability and preventing falls.

This is particularly important for seniors, as balance and stability tend to decline with age.

Furthermore, Marching in Place can be incorporated into a variety of exercise routines. It can serve as a warm-up activity to prepare the body for more intense exercises or be part of a cool-down sequence to gradually lower the heart rate. Its versatility and effectiveness make it a valuable addition to any fitness regimen aimed at improving cardiovascular health and overall physical fitness.

Seated Jumping Jacks are another effective Cardiovascular Chair Exercise that provides a full-body workout while minimizing joint strain. This exercise involves mimicking the motion of traditional jumping jacks but from a seated position. By coordinating arm and leg movements, Seated Jumping Jacks help elevate the heart rate and engage multiple muscle groups simultaneously.

The primary benefit of Seated Jumping Jacks is their ability to provide a high-intensity workout without the need for standing or jumping. This makes them an ideal choice for seniors who may have joint issues or balance concerns. By performing this exercise from a seated position, individuals can enjoy the cardiovascular benefits of traditional jumping jacks without the associated impact on the joints.

Seated Jumping Jacks also promote improved coordination and flexibility. The rhythmic movement of the arms and legs helps enhance motor skills and muscle synchronization, which are crucial for maintaining functional independence. Additionally, this exercise can be modified to suit different fitness levels by adjusting the speed and range of motion.

Incorporating Seated Jumping Jacks into a regular exercise routine can lead to significant improvements in cardiovascular health and overall fitness. Consistent practice can help increase endurance, improve muscle tone, and boost metabolic function. Moreover, this exercise can be performed in various settings, making it a convenient and accessible option for seniors seeking to maintain an active lifestyle.

Arm and Leg Coordination Moves are essential components of Cardiovascular Chair Exercises. These exercises involve simultaneous movements of the arms and legs, promoting improved coordination and muscle synchronization. By engaging multiple muscle groups at once, these moves help elevate the heart rate and enhance cardiovascular endurance.

One of the most effective Arm and Leg Coordination Moves is the seated leg lift combined with arm raises. This exercise involves lifting one leg while raising the opposite arm, then alternating sides. This coordinated movement helps improve balance, enhance coordination, and strengthen the core muscles. Additionally, it provides a cardiovascular workout by increasing the heart rate and promoting better circulation.

Another effective move is the seated bicycle. This exercise involves mimicking the motion of pedaling a bicycle while remaining seated.

By alternating leg movements and incorporating arm swings, this exercise provides a full-body workout that enhances cardiovascular health and improves muscle tone. The seated bicycle is particularly beneficial for seniors as it reduces the risk of joint strain and provides a low-impact alternative to traditional cycling.

Arm and Leg Coordination Moves can be easily modified to suit individual fitness levels. For beginners, the range of motion and speed can be adjusted to ensure comfort and safety.

As fitness levels improve, the intensity can be gradually increased by incorporating resistance bands or weights. This adaptability makes these exercises suitable for a wide range of individuals, from those new to exercise to more advanced participants.

Incorporating Arm and Leg Coordination Moves into a regular fitness routine can lead to significant health benefits. These exercises help improve cardiovascular endurance, enhance muscle tone, and promote better coordination and balance. Additionally, they contribute to overall physical fitness and well-being, making them a valuable addition to any exercise regimen aimed at seniors.

Chair Dancing is a fun and engaging way to improve cardiovascular health while remaining seated. This activity involves performing dance movements from a seated position, incorporating rhythmic arm and leg movements to elevate the heart rate and enhance overall fitness. Chair Dancing is particularly beneficial for seniors as it provides a low-impact alternative to traditional dance workouts, reducing the risk of joint strain and injury.

The primary benefit of Chair Dancing is its ability to provide a full-body workout while being gentle on the joints. By incorporating a variety of dance styles and movements, this exercise helps improve cardiovascular endurance, enhance muscle tone, and promote better coordination. Additionally, Chair Dancing can be performed to a wide range of music, making it a fun way to stay active.

Chair Dancing also offers numerous mental health benefits. The rhythmic movements and music can help reduce stress, improve mood, and promote a sense of well-being.

Additionally, Chair Dancing can be performed in group settings, providing a social component that fosters community and support. This social interaction is particularly important for seniors, as it helps combat loneliness and promotes overall mental health.

Incorporating Chair Dancing into a regular exercise routine can lead to significant improvements in cardiovascular health and overall fitness. Consistent practice can help increase endurance, improve muscle tone, and enhance coordination and balance. Moreover, the enjoyable nature of Chair Dancing makes it a sustainable and engaging way to stay active and healthy.

Low-impact aerobics are an essential component of Cardiovascular Chair Exercises. These exercises involve rhythmic movements that elevate the heart rate while minimizing joint strain. Low-impact aerobics are particularly beneficial for seniors as they provide a way to improve cardiovascular health, enhance endurance, and promote overall physical fitness without the need for high-impact activities.

One of the key advantages of Low-Impact Aerobics is their accessibility. These exercises can be performed from a seated position, making them suitable for individuals with varying levels of mobility and fitness. Additionally, Low-Impact Aerobics can be easily modified to match individual capabilities, ensuring that everyone can participate regardless of their physical limitations.

Low-impact aerobics typically include movements such as arm swings, leg lifts, and seated marches. These exercises help engage multiple muscle groups, promoting improved circulation and enhanced metabolic function. By incorporating rhythmic movements and steady pacing, Low-

Impact Aerobics help elevate the heart rate and improve cardiovascular endurance.

Incorporating Low-Impact Aerobics into a regular fitness routine can lead to significant health improvements. Consistent practice can help reduce the risk of cardiovascular diseases, enhance respiratory function, and improve overall stamina. Additionally, these exercises can contribute to better mental health by reducing stress and promoting a sense of well-being.

Overall, Cardiovascular Chair Exercises, including Marching in Place, Seated Jumping Jacks, Arm and Leg Coordination Moves, Chair Dancing, and Low-Impact Aerobics, provide a safe and effective way for seniors to improve their cardiovascular health and overall physical fitness.

These exercises are accessible, adaptable, and enjoyable, making them an ideal choice for maintaining an active and healthy lifestyle.

CHAPTER 8
Flexibility And Balance Training

Flexibility and balance training are crucial components of chair workouts for seniors.

These exercises focus on improving joint mobility, range of motion, and stability, which are essential for everyday activities and reducing the risk of falls. Chair-based flexibility exercises include gentle stretches targeting major muscle groups such as the legs, arms, back, and neck.

These stretches can be performed seated or standing behind the chair for support, allowing seniors to safely improve their flexibility without straining or overexerting themselves.

Gentle Yoga Poses: Incorporating gentle yoga poses into chair workouts offers numerous benefits for seniors. Yoga promotes flexibility, strength, and relaxation through a series of poses that engage different muscle groups and encourage mindful breathing.

Chair yoga is a modification of basic yoga postures that may be done while seated or with the chair providing support. This allows seniors who struggle with balance or movement to participate in the practice.

Poses, like seated forward, bends, gentle twists and chest openers improve posture, flexibility, and overall well-being.

Tai Chi Movements: Tai Chi is a form of martial arts that is distinguished by deep breathing and gentle, flowing motions.

Chair-based Tai Chi adapts these movements to be performed while sitting or holding onto the chair for support. Tai Chi promotes balance, coordination, and relaxation, making it an excellent addition to chair workouts for seniors. Movements like "Cloud Hands," "Waving Hands Like Clouds," and "Parting Wild Horse's Mane" focus on shifting weight, improving stability, and enhancing mindfulness.

Balance Exercises Using a Chair: Chair-based balance exercises are designed to improve stability and reduce the risk of falls among seniors. These exercises include standing on one leg while holding onto the chair for support, heel-to-toe walking, and side-leg raises while seated. By incorporating balance challenges into chair workouts, seniors can enhance their proprioception, strengthen their lower body muscles, and boost their confidence in performing daily activities safely.

Stretching for Flexibility: Stretching exercises play a vital role in enhancing flexibility and mobility for seniors. Chair workouts can include a variety of stretches targeting different muscle groups, such as hamstring stretches, quadriceps stretches, calf stretches, and shoulder stretches. Stretching improves muscle elasticity, reduces stiffness, and promotes a better range of motion, making everyday movements easier and more comfortable for seniors.

Mindfulness and Relaxation Techniques: Chair workouts for seniors often incorporate mindfulness and relaxation techniques to promote mental well-being and stress reduction. Techniques such as deep breathing exercises, guided imagery, and progressive muscle relaxation can be included in chair-based routines to help seniors unwind, improve focus, and enhance overall relaxation. Mindfulness practices also encourage seniors to be present at the moment, fostering a sense of calmness and tranquility during workouts.

CHAPTER 9
Combining Chair Exercises Into Workouts

Combining chair exercises into workouts for seniors involves strategically selecting exercises that target various muscle groups and movement patterns while considering the limitations and needs of older adults. A key aspect is to include exercises that improve strength, flexibility, balance, and cardiovascular health. For example, incorporating seated leg lifts, arm curls with light weights, and seated marches can improve lower body strength and cardiovascular endurance. Adding in seated side bends, shoulder rolls and neck stretches can enhance flexibility and reduce stiffness. By combining these exercises into a structured routine, seniors can achieve a comprehensive workout that addresses multiple aspects of fitness.

Structuring a Balanced Workout Routine: A balanced workout routine for seniors should include components that address strength, flexibility, balance, and cardiovascular fitness. Structuring such a routine involves planning exercises that target each of these areas while ensuring safety and effectiveness.

For strength, exercises like seated squats, chest presses with resistance bands, and seated rows can be included. Flexibility can be addressed with seated stretches for the hamstrings, shoulders, and hips. Balance exercises such as toe taps, heel raises, and single-leg stands can improve stability. Cardiovascular fitness can be enhanced with seated marches, chair aerobics, or cycling movements. By balancing these components, seniors can maintain overall fitness and improve their quality of life.

Sample Weekly Workout Plans: A sample weekly workout plan for seniors may include a variety of exercises spread across different days to ensure a well-rounded routine. For instance, on Monday, the focus could be on upper body strength with exercises like seated arm curls, shoulder presses, and triceps extensions. Wednesday could be dedicated to lower body strength with seated leg lifts, calf raises, and hip abduction exercises. Friday's workout might emphasize cardiovascular fitness with chair aerobics, seated marches, and arm cycling movements. Throughout the week, flexibility exercises like seated stretches and gentle yoga poses can be incorporated.

This structured approach ensures that seniors work on different aspects of fitness throughout the week while allowing for adequate rest and recovery between sessions.

Modifying Exercises for Different Fitness Levels: Modifying exercises for different fitness levels is essential in chair workouts for seniors to accommodate varying abilities and prevent injury. Beginners may start with lighter resistance or fewer repetitions, gradually increasing intensity as they progress. For those with limited mobility, seated versions of exercises can be used, such as seated leg extensions instead of standing leg lifts. It's important to offer alternatives and adjustments based on individual needs, ensuring that everyone can participate safely and effectively in the workout routine.

Incorporating Rest and Recovery: Incorporating rest and recovery into chair workouts for seniors is crucial for preventing overexertion and allowing the body to repair and strengthen. Adequate rest periods between exercises and workout sessions are essential, as is listening to the body's signals of fatigue or discomfort. Encouraging seniors to hydrate properly, practice deep breathing or relaxation techniques, and get sufficient sleep also supports overall recovery and well-being. By prioritizing rest and recovery, seniors can optimize the benefits of their workout routine and maintain long-term fitness and health.

CHAPTER 10
Adapting Chair Workouts For Specific Conditions

Adapting Chair Workouts for Specific Conditions involves a nuanced approach that considers the unique needs and challenges faced by seniors with various health conditions. One of the key aspects is to ensure exercises are safe, effective, and tailored to address specific issues while promoting overall health and well-being.

For seniors with arthritis, it's crucial to focus on exercises that are gentle on the joints yet help improve flexibility and mobility. Low-impact movements such as seated leg lifts, gentle arm circles, and wrist rotations can be beneficial. Incorporating stretching exercises that target major muscle groups while avoiding excessive strain on the joints is also important. Additionally, using resistance bands or light weights can help strengthen muscles without exacerbating joint pain.

When designing chair workouts for seniors with osteoporosis, the emphasis is on exercises that promote bone health and reduce the risk of fractures. Weight-bearing exercises, even in a seated position, can help maintain bone density. Examples include seated squats, leg extensions, and heel raises. Incorporating balance exercises, such as seated toe taps or heel-toe raises, can also improve stability and reduce the risk of falls.

Cardiovascular health is a critical aspect of overall fitness, even for seniors who may have limited mobility. Chair workouts can be adapted to include cardiovascular exercises that elevate the heart rate and improve circulation. Seated marching or tapping exercises, arm swings, and seated cycling movements can all contribute to cardiovascular fitness. It's important to start at a comfortable pace and gradually increase intensity based on individual fitness levels.

For seniors with limited mobility, chair workouts offer a safe and accessible way to stay active.

Exercises can be modified to accommodate mobility challenges while still providing a full-body workout. Seated exercises that target the upper body, such as shoulder presses, bicep curls, and chest flies, can help maintain muscle strength. Gentle leg exercises like seated leg lifts or knee extensions can also be included to promote lower body mobility.

Pain management is a crucial consideration when designing chair workouts for seniors. Exercises should be chosen carefully to avoid exacerbating existing pain while still providing therapeutic benefits. Incorporating gentle stretches, breathing exercises, and relaxation techniques can help alleviate tension and improve overall comfort. Seniors need to listen to their bodies and adjust the intensity of exercises as needed to avoid discomfort.

By customizing chair workouts to address specific conditions like arthritis, osteoporosis, cardiovascular health, limited mobility, and pain management, seniors can enjoy the benefits of regular exercise in a safe and supportive environment. Consistency, proper form, and gradual progression are key principles to ensure a positive and effective exercise experience for older adults.

CHAPTER 11
Monitoring Progress And Staying Motivated

Monitoring progress and staying motivated are crucial aspects of any fitness program, especially for seniors engaging in chair workouts. Progress monitoring involves tracking various parameters such as strength gains, flexibility improvements, endurance levels, and overall well-being.

It helps individuals understand their journey, identify areas for improvement, and stay motivated to continue their exercise routine. This chapter delves into the importance of monitoring progress and provides strategies for staying motivated throughout the chair workout journey.

Tracking exercise progress is a fundamental component of monitoring progress. Seniors can track their progress through various methods such as keeping a workout journal, using fitness tracking apps, or working with a fitness coach.

By recording details like exercise duration, repetitions, weights used (if applicable), and perceived exertion levels, seniors can gain insights into their progress over time. Tracking progress not only provides tangible data but also serves as a motivating factor by showcasing achievements and highlighting areas of improvement.

Setting realistic goals is essential for seniors embarking on chair workouts. Goals should be specific, measurable, achievable, relevant, and time-bound (SMART). Seniors can set goals related to strength improvements, flexibility gains, cardiovascular endurance, or overall health and well-being. By setting realistic goals, seniors can stay focused, track their progress effectively, and experience a sense of accomplishment as they work towards achieving their objectives.

Overcoming plateaus is a common challenge faced by individuals engaging in any fitness regimen, including chair workouts.

Plateaus occur when progress stagnates, and improvements become less noticeable. Seniors can overcome plateaus by incorporating variety into their workouts, adjusting intensity levels, trying new exercises or techniques, seeking guidance from fitness professionals, and focusing on continuous learning and improvement. Overcoming plateaus requires resilience, patience, and a willingness to adapt and explore new strategies.

Staying consistent and motivated is key to long-term success in chair workouts for seniors. Consistency involves sticking to a regular exercise schedule and making physical activity a part of daily life. Motivation plays a crucial role in sustaining consistency by keeping seniors engaged, enthusiastic, and committed to their fitness goals.

Strategies for staying consistent and motivated include finding enjoyable exercises, setting reminders, enlisting support from friends or family members, joining group fitness classes, rewarding progress, and focusing on the positive impact of exercise on overall health and well-being.

Celebrating milestones is an important aspect of the chair workout journey for seniors. Milestones can include reaching fitness goals, overcoming challenges, improving mobility or functionality, or simply maintaining a consistent exercise routine.

Celebrating milestones reinforces progress, boosts confidence, and provides motivation to continue pushing towards new achievements. Seniors can celebrate milestones by rewarding themselves, sharing successes with others, reflecting on accomplishments, and setting new goals to continue their fitness journey.

Overall, monitoring progress and staying motivated are integral parts of a successful chair workout program for seniors. By tracking progress, setting realistic goals, overcoming plateaus, staying consistent and motivated, and celebrating milestones, seniors can experience the numerous physical, mental, and emotional benefits of regular exercise and maintain a healthy, active lifestyle.

CHAPTER 12
Nutrition And Hydration For Seniors

Nutrition plays a pivotal role in the overall well-being of seniors engaging in chair workouts.

It forms the foundation for their physical health and vitality, influencing their energy levels, recovery, and performance. Proper nutrition becomes even more critical as aging bodies may have different nutrient requirements and metabolic processes. Seniors should prioritize a balanced diet that includes a variety of nutrient-dense foods to support their exercise routine and overall health.

One of the key aspects of proper nutrition for seniors involved in chair workouts is ensuring an adequate intake of macronutrients such as carbohydrates, proteins, and fats. Carbohydrates provide essential energy for workouts and daily activities, while proteins support muscle maintenance and repair, especially important for seniors aiming to preserve muscle mass and strength. Healthy fats, including omega-3 fatty acids, are beneficial for heart health and overall well-being.

In addition to macronutrients, seniors should pay attention to micronutrients like vitamins and minerals. These nutrients play crucial roles in various bodily functions, from immune system support to bone health. Seniors may benefit from incorporating foods rich in calcium, vitamin D, vitamin B12, and antioxidants into their diet. Calcium and vitamin D are particularly important for bone health, helping to maintain bone density and reduce the risk of fractures.

Hydration is another vital aspect of nutrition for seniors engaged in chair workouts. Proper hydration supports overall bodily functions, including circulation, digestion, and temperature regulation. Dehydration can lead to fatigue, cramps, and reduced exercise performance.

Seniors should aim to drink an adequate amount of water throughout the day, especially before, during, and after workouts. Hydration needs may vary depending on factors like exercise intensity, climate, and individual sweat rates.

To optimize their chair workout experience, seniors can follow some hydration tips. These include drinking water regularly throughout the day, not just when feeling thirsty, and choosing water over sugary beverages or excessive caffeine. Electrolyte-rich drinks may be beneficial for longer or more intense workouts, helping to replenish electrolytes lost through sweat.

Pre- and post-workout nutrition is also important for seniors to maximize their exercise benefits and recovery. Before a workout, seniors can consume a light snack or meal containing carbohydrates for energy and a small amount of protein for muscle support. Examples include a banana with yogurt or a whole-grain toast with nut butter.

After a workout, seniors should prioritize a meal or snack rich in protein to aid muscle recovery and repair. This could include a lean protein source like grilled chicken or fish, paired with vegetables and whole grains.

Supplements and vitamins can be a part of a senior's nutrition plan, but they should not replace a balanced diet. Seniors may consider supplements like vitamin D, omega-3 fatty acids, or calcium if they have specific deficiencies or dietary restrictions. However, it's important to consult with a healthcare provider before starting any new supplements to ensure they are safe and appropriate.

The synergy between diet and exercise is undeniable for seniors engaged in chair workouts. A well-rounded diet supports exercise performance, recovery, and overall health outcomes. Regular physical activity, combined with proper nutrition, can help seniors maintain independence, mobility, and a high quality of life.

By paying attention to their nutrition and hydration needs, seniors can optimize their chair workout experience and enjoy the many benefits of staying active and healthy.

Conclusion

Chair workouts for seniors offer a gentle, effective way to stay fit, improve overall health, and maintain independence. The journey begins with understanding the importance of exercise in later years, recognizing the numerous benefits of chair workouts, and ensuring safety throughout each session by setting up a secure workout space.

A fundamental aspect of senior fitness is understanding the common age-related physical changes and assessing individual fitness levels. Setting realistic goals and incorporating medical advice help tailor the workouts to each person's unique needs.

Warm-up and cool-down techniques are essential to prepare the body for exercise and aid in recovery.

Gentle stretching routines, breathing exercises, and proper cool-down strategies ensure a well-rounded approach to each session.

Upper body chair exercises, such as seated arm raises, chair push-ups, shoulder presses, bicep curls, and tricep extensions, target strength and flexibility. Lower body exercises like seated leg lifts, chair squats, calf raise, hamstring curls, and ankle rotations help build lower body strength and stability.

Core strengthening exercises, including seated abdominal twists, chair leg raises, seated side bends, pelvic tilts, and stability ball exercises, are crucial for enhancing core strength and balance. Cardiovascular health is also a focus, with activities such as marching in place, seated jumping jacks, arm and leg coordination moves, chair dancing, and low-impact aerobics.

Flexibility and balance training incorporate gentle yoga poses, Tai Chi movements, balance exercises using a chair, and stretching routines. Mindfulness and relaxation techniques are also introduced to promote mental well-being.

Combining these exercises into balanced workout routines, structuring sample weekly plans, and modifying exercises for different fitness levels ensure inclusivity and adaptability. Rest and recovery are integral parts of maintaining a sustainable fitness regimen.

Specific conditions like arthritis, osteoporosis, cardiovascular issues, and limited mobility require tailored exercises. Pain management is also addressed, ensuring workouts are accessible and beneficial for all.

Monitoring progress, setting realistic goals, and staying motivated are key to long-term success. Tracking progress, overcoming plateaus, and celebrating milestones keep the journey exciting and rewarding.

Nutrition and hydration are vital for seniors, with emphasis on proper nutrition, hydration tips, pre- and post-workout nutrition, and the synergy between diet and exercise. Supplements and vitamins may also play a role in enhancing overall health.

By embracing chair workouts, seniors can enjoy improved physical health, greater independence, and enhanced quality of life.